Siegfried Gursche

*Jennifer
Crawford*

Good
Fats and Oils

Why we need them and
how to use them in the kitchen

D0980699

alive
books
Vancouver
Canada

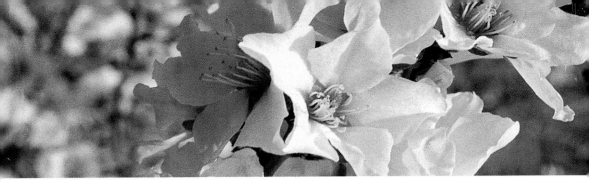

c o n t e n t s

All About Good Fats and Oils

Note: Conversions in this book (from imperial to metric) are not exact. They have been rounded to the nearest measurement for convenience. Exact measurements are given in imperial. The recipes in this book are by no means to be taken as therapeutic. They simply promote the philosophy of both the author and *alive* books in relation to whole foods, health and nutrition, while incorporating the practical advice given by the author in the first section of the book.

Healthy Recipes Using Good Fats and Oils

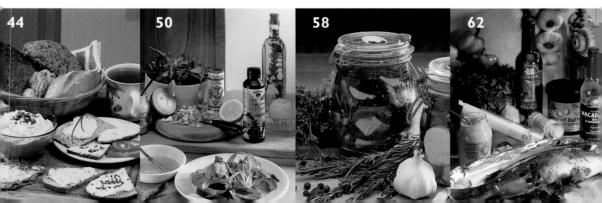

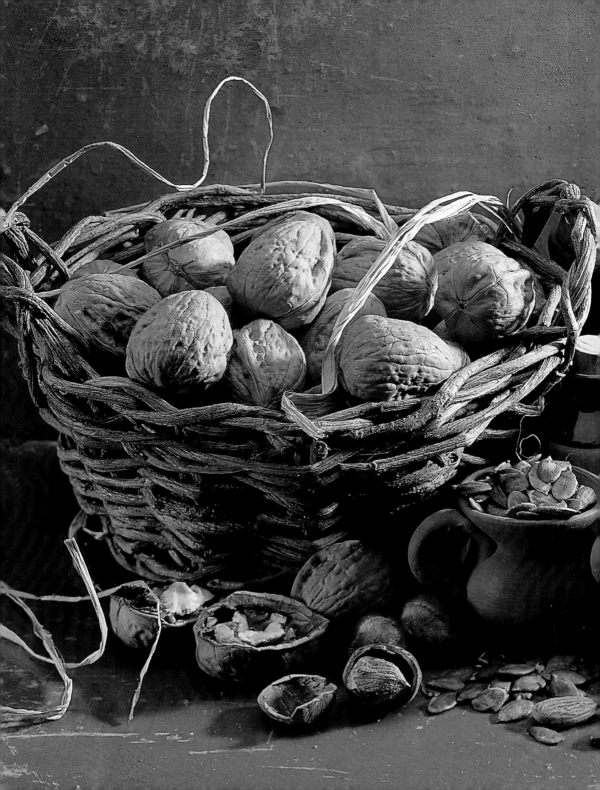

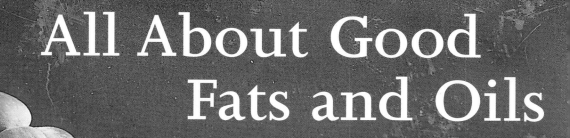

All About Good Fats and Oils

Understanding fats and oils is crucial to your health and to the health of those you love.

Introduction . . . .

In recent years scientists and dietitians have focused on fats to find nutritional answers for the rampant increase of degenerative diseases and the rising tide of obesity. We have been told over and over again that fats are bad for us and we ought to cut down. What we have not been told, however, is that there are many *good* fats and oils.

Here is the irony: The good fats are not only healthy for us but actually help to regulate the entire fat metabolism so that the body systems can function normally. In fact it's the good fats and oils that give us healthy skin, keep our brain and nervous system functioning, prevent cardiovascular disease and even help with weight loss. On the other hand it's true that bad fats cause or contribute to high cholesterol, clogged arteries, obesity and other diseases including cancer. Many people share the misconception that fat is bad. This is not so. In fact, fat is healthy and essential to many life functions. It is one of the three main building blocks of human nutrition (the others are carbohydrates and proteins).

So, which fats are good and which are bad? Why are some okay and others not? How can you make sure you eat good ones and not bad? If you have asked questions like these and been overwhelmed by complex, confusing and conflicting answers instead of simple, practical advice, this book is for you. You will finally understand that butter is healthier than margarine, coconut oil is—in its natural state—one of the best cooking oils available, and that "no-fat" and "low-fat" foods are not healthy options. I will help you understand the differences between good fats and oils and bad ones. More importantly, I will explain how to use good fats and oils to prepare healthful meals.

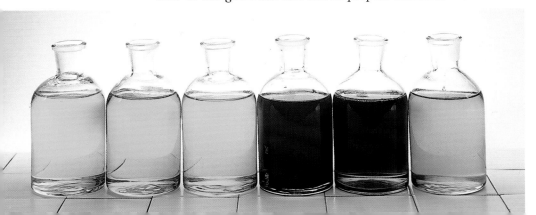

It is not only important to have the knowledge to avoid bad fats and oils and use good ones, but also to know that industrial processing and frying can turn a good fat into a bad, resulting in serious effects to your health. Understanding fats and oils is crucial to your health and to the health of those you love. Recognizing the need to understand fats and oils is the first step toward shopping more wisely and preparing meals that promote health. I will give you the confidence to use the good ones safely and properly for optimum health.

For more information...

Good Fats and Oils is not a scientific rendering and does not cover all aspects of oils and fats in human nutrition. It is a practical guide filled with basic, factual information in straightforward language. For further detail, many books provide scientific information about the roles of oils and fats in health, disease, and nutrition.

In 1955, Dr. Johanna Budwig became the first author to publish information on the role of flax oil in healing cancer and other degenerative diseases. Dr. Budwig has written many books for the scientific community describing the connections between essential fats and vibrant health while warning about the detrimental effects of *trans-fats*. In 1988 Dr. Donald Rudin wrote about the essential fatty acid Omega 3, found in flax oil, and in 1987 Dr. Julius Fast wrote about Omega 3 in fish oils. In 1984, Dr. David Horrobin

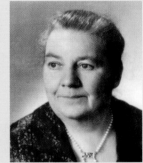
Dr. Johanna Budwig

published his findings on the health benefits of evening primrose oil. Dr. Mary Enig of the University of Maryland continuously publishes scientific papers on *trans-fatty acids*, the worst of the bad fats.

In 1985, *alive* books published a comprehensive book called *Fats and Oils, The Complete Guide to Fats and Oils in Health and Nutrition*, by **Udo Erasmus**. Revised and updated in 1992 as *Fats that Heal-Fats that Kill*, it is now in its eleventh printing, has become a bestseller in English-speaking countries throughout the world, and has been translated into Dutch. To date, no one has written a better book. Its publication was hailed with rave reviews.

A reference book like no other, *Fats that Heal-Fats that Kill* describes the metabolic processing of fat in the human body, because it is only through a thorough understanding of the role of fats and oils in human nutrition that the metabolic process makes sense. However, it wasn't meant to be a practical book providing tips on the use of good fats and oils in the kitchen. The book you are holding will give you the "need to know" information in order to use healthy oils.

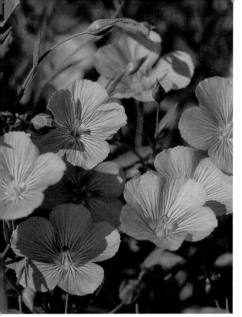

The oil from flax seeds is made up almost entirely of good poly-unsaturated essential fatty acids.

Food: Then and Now . . . .

A century ago, up to one-third of children died in the first two years of life, while older children and adults commonly succumbed to infectious diseases such as tuberculosis, diphtheria, measles and chicken pox, or illnesses related to poor hygiene such as typhoid and diarrhea.

Today, infant mortality in the Western world is low and most diseases that previously threatened human life are well controlled. Yet our generation is plagued with degenerative diseases such as high blood pressure and high cholesterol, and the list is growing. These are diseases that were relative rarities at the turn of century, however, are now rampant and on the increase.

Likewise, the incidences of cancer in the Western world have skyrocketed and obesity is out of control! Where did all this disease come from? How did we get here? It may not be obvious, but today people die mostly from food related degenerative diseases.

Alongside many changes during the past century have been tremendous changes to our food supply. It used to be that foods were produced locally and had short shelf lives. Today most foods are highly processed—designed to travel long distances on transport trucks and sit in grocery stores for a long time without spoiling. Removing the bio-active substances that contribute to quick spoilage stabilizes this designer food. In other words, the nutrition is removed! Why? The answer is sad, but simple. The food industry makes a much larger profit on manufactured, refined and stabilized foods than it would selling the unprocessed, quick spoiling but healthful foods our bodies require.

Our health suffers the consequences. The health of those who consume nutritionally inferior food is not important in such a big business. In the meantime, the more frequently an individual consumes refined food (especially refined oils and processed fats), the more likely that he or she will become ill. In the consumer's mind this food is conceived as normal because part of the profits from selling processed food goes toward advertisements to brainwash them into thinking the food is not only convenient and tasty, but healthy, too.

Millions of dollars are spent to make us believe that we depend on these processed products for our survival and happiness. The exact opposite is true. The more processed food we eat, the sicker we get and the sooner we die. This is especially true for the fats and oils derived from seeds and nuts. In an unrefined state they are health-promoting. Once transformed by refinement, they become disease-promoting.

There is Proof

The health trends we've experienced in Western society are not coincidental. In fact, changes in the health trends of whole populations have been caused by changes in nutrition. This is proven by studies of people who continue to live as their ancestors have for thousands of years.

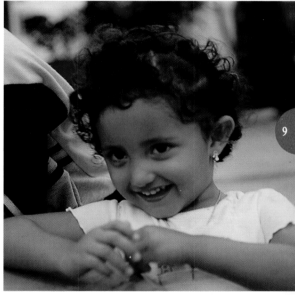

9

In the early 1900s, researchers found that people in isolated villages, on windswept islands or mountainous regions, were much healthier, in many ways, than citizens of industrial societies. Untouched by the eating habits of industrial nations, they had no decaying teeth, heart disease, cancer, hypertension or cholesterol problems. Dr. Weston C. Price, Dr. Francis Pottenger, Dr. Paavo Airola, Dr. John MacDougal and Victor Beguin told amazing stories about the health of tribal peoples living in remote areas.

Changes in the health trends of whole populations have been caused by changes in nutrition.

Among the Saami of Northern Sweden they found people with perfect health–no degenerative cardiovascular disease. Among the indigenous people of Hawaii and other tropical islands, they found no tuberculosis or diabetes. In the Loetschtal valley of Switzerland and among the Hunzas of the Caucasus they found miraculous cases of longevity. Such extraordinary

Refined foods are responsible for today's plagues of degenerative diseases.

health could not be attributed to the "low-fat" or "no-fat" diet fads currently sweeping Western nations in one of the potentially most-damaging nutritional trends ever witnessed.

Dr. Ronald F. Schmidt, author of *Native Nutrition*, and Dr. Henry G. Bieler, author of *Food is Your Best Medicine*, agree: Refined foods are not only detrimental to health, but responsible for today's plagues of degenerative disease. Refined foods include white sugar and flour, commercial and processed vegetable oils, manufactured foods, substances (such as coffee whiteners and artificial sweeteners), and all fractionated foods. Refined and fractionated foods include most of the so-called foods people fill their shopping carts with each week at the grocery store.

The China Project

Beginning in 1983 a collaboration of top universities and scientists from a number of countries, including the US, China, Britain and France, made China into a living laboratory. *The China Project* by T. Colin Campbell and Christine Cox (New Century Nutrition, 1996), is a fascinating account of the results from most comprehensive data base on the multiple causes of disease ever compiled.

China offered perhaps the last place in the world where such a study could be undertaken. Here in the West, we might eat a Honduras-grown banana for breakfast, a Mexican taco for lunch and Italian dish for dinner, followed by a French pastry for dessert. We also tend to move within, and in and out of, our country and continent. However, the Chinese tend to spend their entire lives in the same area and eat the same kinds of locally grown foods throughout their lives.

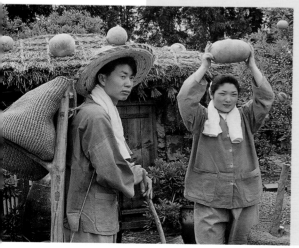

The diets in China vary considerably from one region to another. The scientists wanted to find out if the varying diets in these different regions would correlate to death rates from certain diseases. Their investigations, which were the most widespread and massive scientific investigations ever devised, involved 65 countries and 80 million Chinese. Death rates from specific diseases varied, sometimes several hundredfold from country to country. In relation they estimate that premature deaths from all diseases could be reduced by 80 to 90 percent when the information they found is considered. And guess what? The information is all related to what we eat.

Fats: Then and Now, Here and There . . . .

A correlation between unrefined fats and health, and refined fats and oils (resulting in an increase in the incidence of degenerative disease) has been demonstrated by Dr. Mary Enig, University of Maryland. Her research shows that before 1900, the average person's diet included about 40 percent fats and oils, roughly the same as our diets do today. However, the pre-1900 diet included *unrefined* fats and oils from a variety of sources (animal and vegetable), while today we consume huge amounts of *refined* fats. These fats come to us in the forms of refined liquid oils and artificially hardened fats, such as margarine and shortening, and hidden in much of our processed and fast foods.

What kind of fats are you putting in your shopping cart? And how much? The average Spaniard or Italian consumes 10 liters of olive oil per year, while Libyans consume roughly 20 liters per person per year. Greeks set the global gold standard for olive-oil consumption at 23 liters per person per year, which amounts to about 5 tablespoons of olive oil per day. Other fats are derived from unpasteurized dairy products, such as butter, goat- and sheep-milk cheeses, *laban* (kefir/yogurt), and fish, as well as a small amount of meat.

How does this compare with the amount of fat you consume? Your fats may include butter, margarine, salad and cooking oils, and the hidden fats in meat, baking, and snack foods. By current Western standards, Mediterranean people consume a lot of fat—yet they are legendarily healthy. As Dr. Ancel Keys from the University of Minnesota has shown, the population of Greece has the lowest incidence of heart-related diseases in Europe.

We cannot relate the rise of degenerative disease in Western society to simple over-consumption of fats.

Fat Confusion Today . . . .

I hope that through the information we've covered so far it is clear that we cannot relate the rise of degenerative disease in Western society to simple over-consumption of fats. The facts are obvious, yet many nutrition scientists advise us to reduce fat intake without distinguishing between good and bad fats. No wonder most people are confused and frustrated.

They tell us to avoid saturated fats, which are fats that

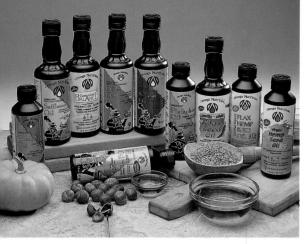

Fats and oils are safe and healthy as long as they are unrefined and neither hydrogenated nor exposed to high temperatures.

normally harden at room temperature (including coconut butter, palm oil and animal fats like suet, lard, and butter). And they tell us that mono- and poly-unsaturated fats (oils that usually remain liquid at room temperature) are good for us. This is extremely misleading! The truth is that neither saturated nor unsaturated fats are bad in their natural states. They are safe and healthy as long as they are unrefined and neither hydrogenated (artificially hardened) nor exposed to high temperature.

Further complicating the issue, orthodox nutrition schools (past and present) typically have classified all foods, including carbohydrates, proteins, fibers and fats, by calories. Calories measure available energy; they cannot, however, measure bio-active substances in food, or secondary nutrients that are essential to the metabolic process and consequently to our well-being. In short, calories really don't count in preserving our health.

It's the nutrients that strengthen our immune systems and prevent the formation of *free radicals*, which cause many degenerative diseases. Sadly, most mainstream nutrition writers ignore such information when presenting nutritional profiles of food. Instead, they focus on caloric values, apparently unaware that oils derived from castor and jojoba beans have no calories at all, and oils from flax seeds and the evening primrose can actually help with weight loss. Good fats don't make you fat!

Good Fats . . . .

In the Western world, we have been taught to believe that eating fat causes us to become fat. So, we think fat is bad for us. As you know already, this is not true. Researchers are only beginning to discover the many good things that fats contribute to health. Fats and oils consist of many different fatty acids that are essential for optimum health. Some fats supply the body with hormone-like substances called *prostaglandins*, which ensure the healthy functioning of many organs. As well, fresh, cold-pressed, unrefined oils contain important elements such as lignans. Although little is known about them, it is already known that they are active in cancer prevention and health promotion.

Lessons from Life

Before the Second World War, my father had a small retail business specializing in butter, hand-made cheeses, butters ground from hazelnuts and almonds, cold-pressed oils and margarine made from non-hardened fats. By that time, hydrogenation, which had been discovered around the turn of the century, had made margarine a cheap and therefore popular alternative to butter. But my father, who as a young man attended lectures by health-food proponents, decided to sell only the best natural products.

One of my father's specialties was a margarine made of natural palm-kernel oil and unrefined coconut butter, both of which naturally harden at room temperature because of their high content of saturated fatty acids. Blended with liquid sunflower oil, this margarine made a spread that was solid yet still spreadable at room temperature. I remember, as a pre-schooler, watching my father open the huge wooden tubs filled with this margarine. I can still smell the fresh aroma when he lifted the protective layer of parchment paper, and savor the taste of the little slivers he gave me.

How quickly those bits melted in my mouth, leaving a slight taste of salt lingering on my tongue! This margarine was different from those we buy in supermarkets today. Because the melting point of the trans-fatty acids (bad fats) in today's margarines is 46°C, it doesn't melt at body temperature, which is 37°C. If you are from my generation you may remember when chocolate used to melt between your fingers if you held it for too long. This was because it was made with natural coconut butter, which melts at 24°C. Today's commercial chocolate deprives us of that sweet pleasure because it melts at a higher temperature. Why? You guessed it: hydrogenated oils with trans-fatty acids.

During my childhood, I learned much about life just by being around and "helping" my father. I learned that fats become rancid quickly when exposed to air. That's why the flax oil my father sold came in metal containers with screw lids: to keep out air. And because refrigeration was not yet common, the containers held just enough to last one week. My father saw his customers weekly, delivering freshly pressed oil made in a village just twenty-five kilometers away. Compare that with the great distances over which food is transported today, and the shelf life foods are expected to have, and it becomes clear how some of these detrimental changes to our food supply have occurred.

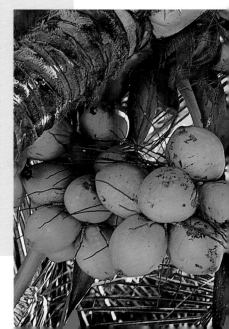

Coconut oil, in its natural state, is one of the best oils for cooking.

Trans-Fatty Acids: Deadly Culprits in Degenerative Disease · · · · · · · · · · · · · · · ·

Hydrogenation is a heat-treatment process used to make liquid oils hard and stabilize them to prevent them from becoming rancid. How? The process removes the bio-active substances that make the oils healthy, because it is these healthy substances that make the oil go rancid (like all natural food eventually does). Removing these substances stabilizes the oils and prevents them from becoming rancid. By adding a hydrogen molecule the liquid becomes hard. This long lasting product (along with promises of health and "low fat") sounds good to the consumer and is therefore an excellent marketing tool. What advertising and food labels don't convey, however, is that the heat process of hydrogenation converts good fatty acids (cis-fatty acids) into harmful fatty acids (trans-fatty acids).

The naturally occurring cis-fatty acids in unrefined oils act as spark plugs in the human body, triggering healthy metabolism of fat. The heat used in the process of hydrogenation transforms cis-fats into trans-fats, which are actually a kind of plastic. With a melting point of 48°C—much higher than human body temperature—our bodies cannot melt trans-fatty acids and therefore cannot metabolize them. In fact, the human body does not even recognize trans-fatty acids as food. Rather, it treats them as toxic elements and seeks dumpsites for them within the body. Dr. Budwig believes cancers are trans-fatty acid deposits.

"European studies have shown that women with breast cancer have higher levels of trans-fats in their tissues than those without the disease."
–Mary G. Enig, PhD

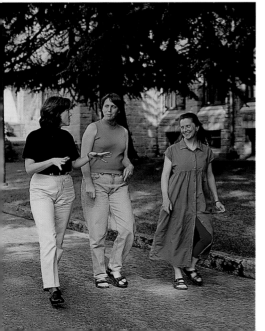

Food manufacturers tell us that trans-fatty acids behave like saturated fats, but in reality they are plastics, which the body cannot metabolize. Trans-fatty acids behave much differently in the human body than cis-fatty acids do. Instead of acting like a spark plug for fat metabolism, trans-fatty acids act more like an ill-fitting ignition key, unable to generate the spark that ignites fat metabolism. Worse, just as that ill-fitting key actually can break off and plug up the system, trans-fatty acids can plug up the liver, preventing the cis-fatty acids your body has absorbed from healthy food sources from performing properly.

In this context, the well-meant advice to reduce total fat consumption makes little sense. A more logical piece of advice would be to eliminate hydrogenated fats from your diet entirely and replace them with untreated natural fats.

It is also important to note that heating oils to extreme temperatures—whether commercially for the purpose of refinement or hydrogenation, or in your own kitchen—changes their molecular structures. A natural, unrefined oil with healthy cis-fatty acids can turn into a bad oil with trans-fatty acids due to heating. Later in the book I will give you specific information about which oils can be heated (and how much) and which cannot.

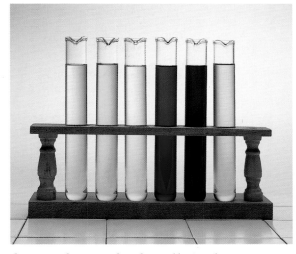

Heating oils to extreme temperatures, whether commercially or while cooking in your kitchen, changes their molecular structures.

Read the Label . . . .

Since the discovery of hydrogenation around the turn of the last century, hardened vegetable oils such as shortening and margarine have been produced and consumed in ever-increasing amounts. Stick margarine is up to 30 percent trans-fatty acids while shortening is up to 50 percent of these bad fats. But hardened fats are not the only problem. Most oils sold in supermarkets are heat-refined, too. Most commercial baked products, including breads, cookies, cakes, packaged foods, candy bars and chocolate, contain 30-50 percent trans-fatty acids, as do commercial salad dressings, potato chips and fried fast foods. These fats are usually declared on the label as modified or partially hydrogenated vegetable oil or vegetable oil shortening.

For your health's sake, and for the sake of your family's health, become a label-reader. Choose virgin or extra virgin olive oil, or other cold-pressed, unrefined oils for cooking. Dip your bread in olive oil, as they do in Mediterranean countries, instead of spreading it with margarine. Check ingredients lists before buying packaged foods, and reject products made with modified fats and hydrogenated oils.

> Artificially harden fats (bad fats) are listed on food labels as *hydrogenated, modified, fractionated* or *partially hydrogenated vegetable oil*. Avoid all products that contain these dangerous fats.

Food Manufacturers usually use inexpensive oils that are unpalatable in their unrefined state, such as cottonseed, palm, canola or soya oil. Adding to the fact that these processed oils have been turned into bad fats, they are also usually made from genetically engineered vegetable oils. Thus, product manufacturers choose cheap, poor-tasting ingredients and refine them to improve their taste, at the same time converting good cis-fats to bad trans-fats. They then enjoy their profits at the expense of your health.

The Government is Not on Your Side

Not only is the government allowing manufacurers to make money at the cost of your health, but they are allowed to do this without a clear indication on the product label of what they have done. Why? Because Canadian Food Labeling legislation does not require trans-fatty acids to be listed on food labels.

When Canadian food labeling underwent changes in the late 1980s, I called Dr. Margaret Cheney at the Health Protection Branch of Health and Welfare Canada in Ottawa and suggested that trans-fatty acids be shown on labels. She replied that consumers wouldn't understand the term and that it wouldn't be in the interest of industry. Instead, trans-fatty acids are included on labels under the general category of saturated fats. But as we have discussed, this is seriously misleading.

But times are changing. Many consumers, such as you, are becoming aware of and concerned about trans-fatty acids. The Food and Drug Administration (FDA) in the US has come under extreme pressure from public interest groups to change nutrition labels on packaged foods so that they list trans-fatty acids separately. Of course, oil and food producers and packagers oppose this as they well know that consumer awareness could affect their profits as negatively as their products could affect our health.

Cholesterol in the Cross-Fire

Many people avoid the wonderful tastes of different natural cheeses and butter because of misinformation about fat and concern about cholesterol content. Similarly, many health-conscious people have dared not eat eggs for years, because they have been taught that eggs are high in cholesterol and can contribute to obesity and heart attacks. The cholesterol scare arose from a study conducted in the 1930s of people who consumed large quantities of dried-egg powder. Dried-egg powder contains oxidized fat. Oxidized fat is rancid fat. It is not the eggs that raise cholesterol, but the rancid fat. Dr. Kurt Donsbach demonstrated this in a study of students who consumed ten fresh boiled eggs per day for thirty days with no increase in cholesterol levels.

There is no need to be confused by cholesterol. The human body makes its own cholesterol and, under normal circumstances, controls the level. Usually 20 percent of cholesterol in the body comes from food, while the body produces 80 percent. If food intake supplies too little cholesterol, the body will make the cholesterol it requires. However, ingesting bad fats, like saturated beef fat and trans-fatty acids, triggers the liver to produce more cholesterol than the body requires. This shows up in the blood stream as elevated cholesterol.

Today, scientists look at cholesterol more favorably. They understand the difference between good cholesterol–high-density lipoproteins or HDL–and bad cholesterol–low-density lipoproteins or LDL. The body needs HDL to produce hormones, bile and Vitamin D. It's also essential to the structuring of cell membranes and proper brain functioning.

To understand the functioning of HDL and LDL, picture them as little trucks loaded with cholesterol. The LDL carries cholesterol through the bloodstream to construction sites. When the liver produces too much cholesterol, the LDL tries to carry bigger loads. The problem is that it loses some along the way, which then sticks to the walls of the arteries. This causes the arteries to narrow, making it more and more difficult for blood to flow freely. This makes the heart work harder, which causes hypertension. But HDL trucks, on the other hand, pick up the excess cholesterol spilled by the overloaded LDL trucks. The HDL trucks carry this excess back to the liver, which expels it with bile into the intestines. Fiber from food we ingest then acts like a brush cleaning out the cholesterol from the intestine, which is one of the reasons for consuming a diet that's high in fiber.

Eggs do not raise cholesterol.

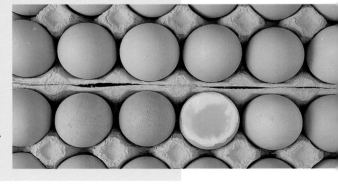

Good Fats Make Good Food . . . .

High-quality oils can enhance the flavor of even the simplest meal. A friend of mine, a famous chef in Austria, taught me that it is impossible to prepare a good, healthy meal with the cheap, refined oils usually found on supermarket shelves. A good meal starts with a high-quality oil and can provide the most wonderful taste in the world.

The best way to learn about oils is to sample different kinds. Oils not only look and taste different but each has its own character as well. Because our government does not require oils to be labeled "refined" or "unrefined," it's impossible for the unaware consumer to know their quality. Natural, unrefined oils such as pumpkinseed, flax, walnut, hazelnut and olive oil are darker in color than refined oils, and have distinctive flavors.

The best places to find unrefined, cold-pressed oils are culinary-specialty shops and health-food stores. But be aware that many health-food stores carry both refined and unrefined oils. Extra virgin olive oil is the only unrefined oil consistently found in supermarkets and delicatessens. Look for natural unrefined oils and use the information in this book to use them confidently when preparing healthful, tasty meals for you and your family. Your taste buds will be happy and your body will be healthy.

Good Oils for Good Fat . . . .

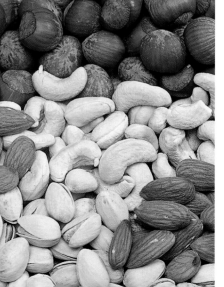

Traditionally, people have found the fats they needed in locally grown seeds, nuts, kernels, fruits, fish, fowl and animals. Whatever the source, it provided a fat or oil with a profile that met the nutritional requirements of the indigenous population. People living in colder climates, where the blood needs to be more liquid, require more poly-unsaturated fatty acids like omega-3 and omega-6. The Inuit and Innu of Canada's North get omega-3 from fish oil. People from less remote but still cold climates get these substances from the oils of seeds and nuts that like a colder environment, like flax, pumpkin, and sunflower seeds, and walnuts.

In a more moderate climate, people flourish on mono-unsaturated fatty acids like Omega 9, which is plentiful in olive oil, pistachio, hazelnut, almond, sesame and avocado oils. In tropical countries, with their abundant sunlight and warmth, the main fat sources are oils rich in saturated fats, some of which harden at room temperature, like coconut, palm and palm-kernel oil. Also rich in saturated fats are oils derived from brazil and macadamia nuts, as well as oil from peanuts (which are actually legumes) and soya beans.

For culinary purposes, I prefer natural nut and seed oils. Different kinds of oils can be mixed to prevent the strong flavor of an individual oil from dominating. For example, I sometimes mix olive and flax oils, or flax and pumpkinseed oils. Almond oil gives a neutral but flavorful addition to a meal.

Know and Avoid Unhealthy Oils . . . .

There are many food oils available commercially, but most have been extracted with the chemical hexane and must be refined to make them palatable. Personally, I join those nutritionists in the whole-foods movement who considers refined oils a "dead food" lacking in vital elements. These are the oils usually found in supermarkets, which include refined safflower, peanut, cottonseed, soya, grapeseed, canola (also known as rapeseed), and even the "light" olive oils.

You also need to watch out for the oils that have been cleverly marketed. "Olivera," for example sounds like an olive oil, but it is actually refined canola oil. Likewise, "light" olive oil is actually refined oil, but consumers might think that "light" refers to fewer calories. These oils are highly processed and have a significant trans-fatty acids content. As well, margarine and vegetable shortening have no place in a whole-foods kitchen.

Let's Get Specific . . . .

It's time to discuss the specifics of good fats and oils and how to safely use them in your kitchen. The following information is invaluable and, if taken to heart and practiced, will forever increase good health and decrease the likelihood of suffering from one of the many degenerative diseases that plagues our society today. While health results from more than just eating healthy oils, this knowledge, along with a balanced life that includes exercise and whole foods diet, will make a significant difference.

Butter is Better

Butter is a good fat. It's a much healthier choice than processed margarines that, for the most part, contain trans-fatty acids. Butter has been a healthy staple throughout history and should still be today. An excreted fat of animal origin, it should not be confused with meat fat. It consists not only of saturated fats, as is generally believed. It also contains good, mono-unsaturated fatty acids and even traces of the essential fatty acids our bodies need to be healthy.

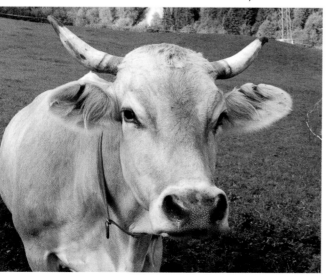

Butter is easily digested without putting any stress on the liver. According to Dr. Alfred Vogel of Switzerland, one of the pioneers the natural health movement, a healthy liver can metabolize 2 heaping tablespoons (60 grams) of butter daily without any special exercise. In general, the body can metabolize 1 gram of butter per kilogram of body weight. To tranpose pounds into kilograms, divide the number of pounds of by 2.2. In other words, a person who weighs

180 pounds weighs roughly 81 kilograms and can metabolize 1 gram of butter per kilogram or roughly 80 grams of butter per day.

If butter is so valuable in human nutrition, why does it have such a poor reputation? Butter was demonized by margarine and shortening manufacturers. Their goal was to change consumer's buying habits in order to gain a bigger market share, and it worked. They had help achieving this goal by medical doctors who do not study nutrition as a part of their training and believed the industry's advertising.

Composition of Butter	
Saturated fatty acids:	Mono-unsaturated fatty acid:
7 % capric acid	24 % buteric acid
2 % lauric acid	Poly-unsaturated fatty acids:
8 % myristic acid	3 % linoleic acid (Omega 6)
21 % palmitic acid (Omega 7)	4 % Other fatty acids
10 % stearic acid (Omega 9)	
2 % others	

Kitchen tips for butter

Have no fear—butter is a good fat. It can be used for baking, frying and cooking, as long as the heat is kept low enough to prevent burning. When butter is heated too much it will burn, just like any other fat, and turn brown. If you accidentally burn butter you've turned good fat into bad, creating trans-fatty acids, so throw the butter away and start again.

Eggs can be fried in butter on low heat, as long as neither the eggs nor the butter turn brown. It's a good idea to use some water-containing vegetables such as onions, potatoes or a mixture of vegetables for stir fries when frying with butter, as they help to prevent it from burning. When preparing other vegetables, it is best to steam them and add butter just before serving. Butter enhances the flavor of any meal.

Olive Oil

Health-conscious gourmets, nutritionists and scientists praise the benefits of olive oil, which is considered by many to be "the queen among oils," as it intensifies the flavor of any dish while promoting health. It is important to understand the quality differences and grading of olive oil. Much as the production of great wines depends on the type of grape, growing conditions, harvesting methods and production techniques. Much in the same way the quality and flavor of olive oil depends upon the type of tree, constituency of soil, climate conditions, harvesting methods and pressing techniques.

Greece, where the olive tree originated, boasts the highest per capita consumption of olive oil in the world, with the average person consuming 23 liters per year. Seventy-three percent of olive oil produced in Greece is consumed within the country. Eight-hundred million olive trees grow throughout the world, 600 million of them in Mediterranean nations. Each mature tree yields about 300 kilograms of olives, enough for 65 liters of oil. Most Mediterranean countries, including Israel, Libya, Tunisia, Turkey, Morocco, Algeria and Syria, export little olive oil. Italy, Spain, Portugal, and Greece are the largest exporters. Still, olive oil comprises only 5 percent of total vegetable-oil consumption throughout the world.

Generally, French olive oil has a light taste, because the French growing regions are less sunny than those further south. Spain and Portugal produce oils that are yellow and heavy. Spain is the world leader in olive-oil production, much of which is exported. Greek olive oils have a pronounced green color and a medium weight. Price-wise, they offer the best value. Italian oils have the greatest variety of flavors and colors, tending more toward green than yellow. The best oils in the world are

Olive oil is still produced by a centuries-old method in many parts of the world such as Isreal.

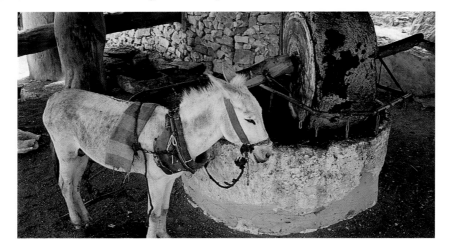

organically grown on private estates, hand picked and carefully processed. Of course, these oils are highly priced, seldom exported and hard to find in North America.

Instead you will find a large variety of excellent olive oils produced in California by small farms. Many Californian olive oil producers have decided to grow organic olives, according to Californian law. Your health food store will know who these suppliers are and will be able to bring you quality oils from this area.

The expression "cold-pressed" to describe oil production comes, not surprisingly, from the fact that the oil is produced without heat being applied externally or generated internally. When I traveled in Israel, I witnessed a centuries-old method of olive-oil production first hand. The ripe olives are hand picked or shaken off the trees and gathered into nets. They are then taken to a mill where the pits are removed and the olives are crushed into a paste. The paste is thickly spread onto fiber mats, which are stacked up in layers in a press. The pressure applied is not too great in order to avoid heat from building up. The oil that comes out of the press is a dark reddish-green. In earlier days, this oil was stored in large containers until the sediment settled. These days, the sediment is cleared out with a centrifuge.

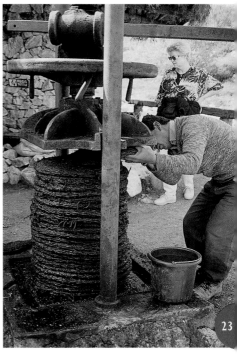

"Cold-pressed" olive oil is produced without heat being applied externally or generated internally.

So many choices

The first pressing produces an olive oil of perfect flavor and aroma with a light yellow to green color. If the acidity is not more than 1 percent, it is graded as *extra virgin olive oil*. The second pressing, where more pressure is applied, still produces an oil of perfect flavor, aroma and color, but with an acidity of 1.5-3.3 percent. This oil is graded as *virgin olive oil*.

Once heat is applied, the resulting oil is slightly less flavorful and has an acidity of more than 3.3 percent. This is called *pure olive oil*. The remaining mash is subjected to a chemical extraction method with hexane or butane and produces oil that must be refined. It is light in color and bland in taste, and is most often labeled *olive oil*, *light olive oil*, or even *olive oil-extra light*.

For health and taste, it makes sense to purchase the best quality. Unrefined virgin olive oil contains traces of many minerals, among them magnesium, potassium and calcium.

Health Benefits of Unrefined Virgin Olive Oil

- prevents heart and circulatory diseases
- prevents hypertension and increases blood fluidity
- increases good (HDL) cholesterol and decreases bad (LDL) cholesterol
- provides protection against cholesterol deposits
- lowers glycemic index of foods and prevents obesity
- supplies antioxidants, protects from free radicals and helps prevent cancer
- emollient effect protects against ulcers
- stimulates bile secretion, promotes gall flow and reduces risk of gallstones
- strengthens liver functions and aids in fat metabolism
- stimulates digestion, aids in passage of food and prevents constipation
- feeds the brain and nervous system
- builds strong bones and prevents osteoporosis
- soothes joint pain and acts as an anti-arthritic agent
- smoothes skin irritations, acts as anti-inflammatory agent
- improves healing by acting as an antibacterial agent and disinfectant

Composition of Olive Oil

Vitamin E and provitamin A (carotene)
Fat Profile - average
78	% mono-unsaturated fatty acids (mainly oleic - Omega 9)
11	% saturated fatty acids (mainly palmitic - Omega 7; a little stearic - Omega 9)
11	% poly-unsaturated fatty acid (linoleic - Omega 6)
0.5	% poly-unsaturated fatty acid (linolenic - Omega 3)

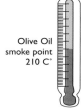

Olive Oil
smoke point
210 C°

Physical Properties of Olive Oil

Solidification point	2°C	Smoke point	210°C
Melting point	5-7°C	Weight	1 liter = 912 grams

24

Kitchen tips for olive oil

Since olive oil consists of mostly mono-unsaturated (omega-9) and saturated fatty acids (palmitic), it can be used in cold dishes as well as for cooking and baking. In an experiment at the University of Bologna in Italy, olive oil was boiled for two hours at 102°C (apx. 215°F). No changes in the fat profile were observed, and no trans-fatty acids were created.

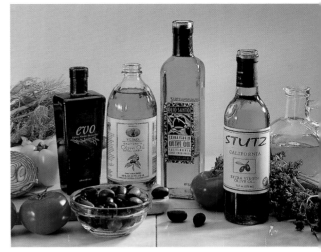

California offers a variety of good quality olive oils.

Olive oil is good when baking bread because the temperature within the loaf is kept below 100°C. However, it's wise to take care when frying with olive oil; keep the temperature below the smoke point, and always add onions or other water-containing vegetables to stir-fries cooked in olive oil. In gourmet kitchens, most fat used to enhance flavor is added *after* the food has been cooked. See the recipe section for great suggestions.

Flax Oil

Flax oil is in a class of its own because it is the only oil comprised almost entirely of good, poly-unsaturated, essential fatty acids. Essential fatty acids are those required by the body to sustain health. These fatty acids must come from food sources because the body cannot produce them. Poly-unsaturated oils are "hungry" for oxygen, which is why they go rancid quickly. This is also why linseed oil (linseed is another name for the seed of the flax plant) is used in paint: Its oxygen-soaking ability causes it to dry quickly.

Flax seeds are 42 percent oil. When expeller-pressed in a cold process, the yield is about 33 percent oil. This oil is 48-64 percent linolenic fatty acid or Omega 3 (LNA), making flax the richest plant source of this nutrient. It is 16-34 percent linoleic fatty acid or Omega 6 (ALA). Of the balance, about 18 percent is oleic fatty acid or Omega 9, a mono-unsaturated but not essential fatty acid.

The Flax Comeback

Flax oil fell out of favor for a number of years, until Dr. Johanna Budwig initiated a comeback. She created the now famous oil-protein diet for patients suffering from cancer, cardiovascular disease, arthritis and other degenerative conditions. The recipe she created consisted mainly of flax oil mixed with quark (a soft, spreadable cheese made by straining warmed-up kefir, yogurt or buttermilk), a grated apple and freshly ground flax seeds. (See recipe section for the "Budwig Muesli.")

Dr. Budwig maintains that fresh, unrefined flax oil has the best health-giving profile for human consumption, provided that it is not heated. Heating poly-unsaturated fats turns good cis-fatty acids into bad trans-fatty acids. It is now widely accepted that trans-fatty acids are the culprits in certain cancers, heart disease and many other degenerative diseases.

When choosing flax oil—as with any edible oil—exercise caution. Not all manufacturers offer high-quality products or deliver what they promise on their product labels. Labels often read "cold-pressed" or "expeller-pressed," hiding the fact that the oil has been refined after extraction. No legislation is in place to make companies disclose that their product has been refined.

Cold-pressed, unrefined, fresh flax oil was first commercially produced in North America only in 1984. It is pressed in small volumes, at temperatures of 45°C or less. With proper packaging that excludes light and oxygen, it can stay fresh for up to six months. On the label, look for a statement that includes the words "cold expeller-pressed" and, most importantly, "unrefined." Also look for a pressing date, and do not purchase flax oil more than six months past this date.

Do not heat flax oil. Use it in cold dishes or on cooked food only.

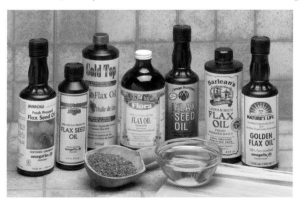

With flax oil, it's better to buy the smaller size bottle to ensure it will be used up within the safe amount of time. At least six reliable companies in Canada and the US press flax oil the way it should be done. These oils can be found only in health food stores and are listed in the "Sources" section at the back of this book.

Health Benefits of Flax Oil

- normalizes the body's fatty acids, resulting in smoother, healthier skin, shiny hair and soft hands
- normalizes blood fats and increases blood fluidity, prevents blood platelets from sticking together and reduces hypertension
- prevents heart and circulatory diseases by decreasing bad (LDL) cholesterol
- normalizes, re-balances and supports prostaglandins, elevates estrogen levels in blood, alleviates adverse symptoms of (PMS) and menopause, and regulates sex hormones
- stabilizes insulin and blood-sugar levels, preventing high-low sugar blues
- corrects the body's thermogenic system by burning fat (ability to burn off calories)
- supports liver functions, aids in fat metabolism, slows down glucose absorption and thus helps with weight loss
- feeds the brain and nervous system and reduces stress
- supplies antioxidants, protects from free radicals and helps prevent cancer
- stimulates the immune system

Composition of Flax Oil

Vitamin E and provitamin A (carotene)
Fat Profile - average
58 % poly-unsaturated fatty acids (linolenic - Omega 3)
19 % poly-unsaturated fatty acids (linoleic - Omega 6)
18 % mono-unsaturated fatty acid (oleic - Omega 9)
 4 % saturated fatty acid (palmitic - Omega 7)
 1 % saturated fatty acid (stearic - Omega 9)

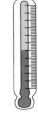

Flax Oil
smoke point
112 C°

Physical Properties of Flax Oil

Solidification point	-22°C	Weight	1 liter = 912 grams
Melting point	-18°C	Color	golden yellow
Smoke point	112°C		

Kitchen tips for flax oil

Since flax oil is poly-unsaturated, with the main component being Omega 3, it spoils quickly when heated or exposed to oxygen and light. Use it in cold dishes only, such as dressings for

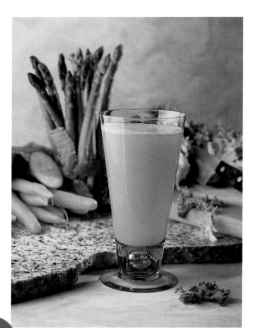

all kinds of green salads, potato salad, grated-carrot salad, coleslaw or raw sauerkraut, or even with kefir and quark. You may want to check all cold recipes calling for oil as an ingredient and see whether flax oil can be used as an alternative. Dips made with quark, yogurt or kefir can be improved nutritionally with the addition of flax oil. Delicious and healthy spreads using butter or coconut butter can be made with flax oil. Check the recipe section for ideas.

Flax oil should not be used for cooking or frying, but you can drizzle it over cooked food. I enjoy dipping freshly baked rye bread in flax oil. It's also delicious when poured over a baked potato and topped with some herbal seasoning. If you are a fan of green drinks or you press your own carrot juice, stir 1 tablespoon of flax oil into a tall glass.

Adding 1 tablespoon of flax oil to a glass of juice makes a healthy combination.

Although many people are not excited about the flavor of flax oil the first time they try it, it is an oil your taste buds can get used to. In fact, you may get hooked! And keep in mind that flax oil is both medicine and food. Two tablespoons per day is just enough.

Pumpkinseed Oil

This oil may never be popular with those seeking a bright golden color and neutral taste, but gourmets and whole-foods enthusiasts treasure its distinct flavor and medicinal value. Its pleasant, nutty-sweet taste makes pure pumpkinseed oil a gourmet salad oil like no other. This is why professional chefs worldwide treasure this precious oil, while nutritionists know that pumpkinseed oil is an excellent healing oil.

The pumpkin's origins have been traced to southern Mexico, where 10,000 years ago indigenous peoples nibbled on the seeds. The oil-bearing seeds with their high protein content were staples of Aztecan and Mayan diets. Pumpkins made their way to Europe in 1492 on Columbus' return voyage, and 180 years later written instructions for growing pumpkins and extracting oil from their seeds were published in Austria. To this day, the Austrian region of Steiermark is the major growing and production area for pumpkinseed oil.

Nutritionally, unrefined pumpkinseed oil is a highly prized and valuable whole food as well as an effective *nutraceutical* (a food with healing properties). However, this is true only as long as the oil is cold-pressed and unrefined. Applying heat to the kernels until they are slightly roasted yields more oil than pressing the seeds cold with a hydraulic press, and for this reason pure, cold-pressed pumpkinseed oil is fairly expensive.

Oil manufacturers often mix cheaper, heat-processed pumpkinseed oil with another low-priced oil, such as sunflower-seed or rapeseed oil, to keep the price down while still calling it pumpkinseed oil. You can test the oil yourself for purity. One drop of genuine pumpkinseed oil on a lettuce leaf will remain a solid drop, while mixed oil will disperse easily.

Unrefined pumpkinseed oil is valuable for both its nutritional and healing properties.

The higher cost of genuine, pure, pumpkinseed oil is justified by its legendary healing properties. Millions of people suffer from bladder weakness or incontinence. Pumpkinseed oil is the best natural remedy for incontinence. Dr. Rudolf F. Weiß, professor of phytotherapy at Freie Universität Berlin, is convinced that pumpkinseed oil is an effective biological medicine for the urinary tract.

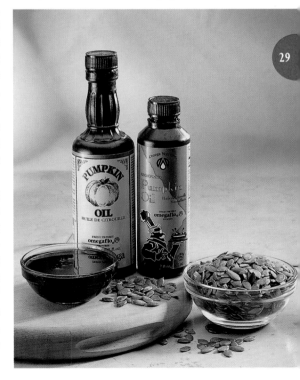

Pumpkinseed oil also has a long reputation for preventing prostate enlargement. This condition occurs when testosterone becomes concentrated in the cells of the prostate. Recent clinical studies confirm that a unique medicinal ingredient called *Delta 7 sterole*, which is found in large amounts in pumpkinseeds and its unrefined oil, can prevent this hormonal build-up from occurring.

Health Benefits of Pumpkinseed Oil

- beneficial for healthy functioning of the prostate gland
- protects from free radicals, supplies antioxidants and helps prevent cancer
- normalizes, re-balances and supports prostaglandins, elevates estrogen levels in the blood, alleviates adverse symptoms of PMS and menopause, and regulates sex hormones
- normalizes blood fats and increases blood fluidity, prevents blood platelets from sticking together and reduces hypertension
- prevents heart and circulatory diseases by decreasing bad (LDL) cholesterol
- influences the body's thermogenic system, burns off fat (ability to burn off calories) and helps in weight loss
- supports liver functions, aids in fat metabolism and slows down glucose absorption
- feeds the brain and nervous system, activates learning ability and reduces stress
- stimulates the immune system

Composition of Unrefined Pumpkinseed Oil

2-4 % vital components including sterols
Fat Profile - average
12 % poly-unsaturated fatty acids (linolenic - Omega 3)
40 % poly-unsaturated fatty acids (linoleic - Omega 6)
29 % mono-unsaturated fatty acid (oleic - Omega 9)
17 % saturated fatty acid (mainly palmitic - Omega 7)
 2 % saturated fatty acid (stearic - Omega 9)

Pumpkinseed Oil smoke point 112 C°

Physical Properties of Unrefined Pumpkinseed Oil

Solidification point	-1°C	Weight	1 liter = 912 grams
Melting point	2-3°C	Color	dark reddish-green
Smoke point	112°C		

Kitchen tips for pumpkinseed oil

Pumpkinseed oil has a distinct aroma and nutty flavor. It improves the taste of salads, gravies, vegetable sauces, pasta and even rice. See the recipe section for sauces and gravies. As with flax oil, only use pumpkinseed oil cold or drizzled over a cooked meal.

Walnut Oil

A highly nutritional oil makes up about one half of the walnut. This oil is easily extracted and has been used for culinary purposes for over 1,000 years. Walnut oil is rich in linoleic acid (omega-6), which produces prostaglandins, a hormone-like substance that's beneficial to the sex organs. Historically, walnut oil has been recommended to increase fertility in women. Check the label before purchasing walnut oil. Some European imports are often refined, with a bland flavor, light color and a fair amount of trans-fatty acids.

Although walnut trees are native to Asia, they are now grown in Middle and Southern Europe and North and South America as well. The US is the largest producer of walnuts in the world today. Friends of mine are the proud owners of a large walnut grove in the Fraser Valley near Vancouver, BC. They are their own best customers, and the healthiest people you can imagine, who provide living proof that consuming large amounts of walnuts regularly does not make people gain weight; they provide healthy fat the body can use.

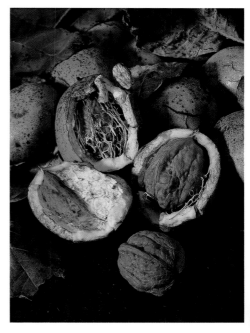

31

Walnut oil has a unique taste and wide range of health benefits.

Health Benefits of Unrefined Walnut Oil

- prevents heart and circulatory diseases by decreasing bad (LDL) cholesterol and increasing good (HDL) cholesterol
- reduces hypertension and normalizes blood fats
- supports production of prostaglandins and regulates sex hormones
- plays a role in the body's thermogenic system, helps control fat metabolism (ability to burn off calories) and body weight
- feeds the brain and nervous system and reduces stress
- supplies antioxidants, protects from free radicals and helps prevent cancer
- stimulates the immune system

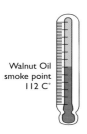

Walnut Oil
smoke point
112 C°

Composition of Unrefined Walnut Oil
Contains Vitamin A, B and E
Fat Profile-average
16 % poly-unsaturated fatty acids (linolenic - omega-3)
59 % poly-unsaturated fatty acids (linoleic - omega-6)
16 % mono-unsaturated fatty acid (oleic - omega-9)
9 % saturated fatty acid (mainly palmitic - omega-7)

Physical Properties of Unrefined Walnut Oil			
Solidification point	-2°C	Weight	1 liter = 912 grams
Melting point	1-3°C	Color	light yellow
Smoke point	112°C		

Kitchen tips for walnut oil

The epicurean quality of walnut oil depends largely upon the quality of the nuts themselves, which can vary tremendously. Walnut oil, when cold pressed and unrefined, is a special addition to the whole-foods kitchen. It enhances fine salads and gives carrots and other root vegetables a palatable, sensual flavor. Walnut oil must not be heated, but can be added to warm dishes after cooking. A mayonnaise made with only natural ingredients and unrefined walnut oil (see page 56) is a fabulous taste experience.

Hemp Oil

Hemp oil provides an excellent balance of essential fatty acids.

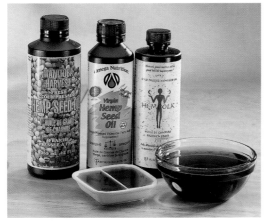

There has been much talk recently about hemp oil, simply because it is a very nutritious oil with an excellent balance of essential fatty acids. Some nutritionists claim that the ratio between linolenic acid (omega-3) and linoleic acid (omega-6) is nothing short of ideal. Hemp oil even contains the rare gamma-linoleic acid (GLA). Udo Erasmus (author of *Fats that Heal-Fats that Kill*, *alive* books, 1992) calls it the twin sister to flax oil because it shares the same health claims. Hemp, however, belongs to the *cannabis* family and is related to marijuana. That's why hemp growing was severely restricted until recently, although hemp seeds contain no hallucinogens.

Composition of Unrefined Hemp Oil

Fat Profile - average
19 % poly-unsaturated fatty acids (linolenic - Omega 3)
57 % poly-unsaturated fatty acids (linoleic - Omega 6)
13 % mono-unsaturated fatty acid (oleic - Omega 9)
  6 % saturated fatty acid (palmitic - Omega 7)
  2 % saturated fatty acid (stearic - Omega 9)
  2 % GLA (gamma-linoleic acid)

Kitchen tips for hemp oil

Unrefined, cold-pressed hemp oil has a fresh, nutty flavor. Because it is rich in essential fatty acids, hemp oil should not be heated. It is pricey, and therefore you may want to use it in combination with olive oil in Greek salads, hummus and marinated foods. This gives you a perfect fat profile. Use it alone, and cold, on baked potatoes and cooked-vegetable salads, and in smoothies.

Hazelnut Oil

A plant native to Europe and used by humans as early as the Stone Age, the hazelnut has been popular for snacks and nut butters for centuries. During the Middle Ages, hazelnuts had such a reputation for curing impotence that Hildegard von Bingen demonized them for their voluptuary attributes. Hazelnuts contain 65 percent oil of which 12 percent is Omega 6, metabolized by the body into prostaglandins, which exert a healthy influence on the sexual organs. Hazelnut oil is also treasured for cosmetic purposes and as a massage oil.

Hazelnut oil is delicate and pleasant tasting, but has a strong and penetrating smell. Produced for culinary purposes only since 1975, it has become popular quickly among leading chefs as an exquisite salad oil.

Hazelnut oil can withstand moderate heat and therefore be used as a baking ingredient.

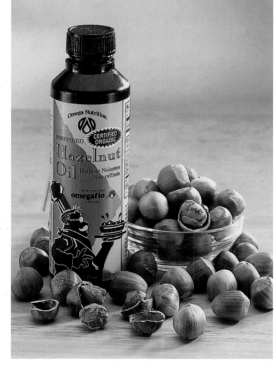

Composition of Hazelnut Oil
Fat Profile - average
76 % mono-unsaturated fatty acids (mainly oleic)
10 % saturated fatty acids (mainly palmitic - omega-7; a little stearic - omega-9)
12 % poly-unsaturated fatty acid (linoleic - omega-6)
2 % poly-unsaturated fatty acid (linolenic - omega-3)

Kitchen tips for hazelnut oil

Since hazelnut oil withstands moderate heat, it can be used for baking nut cakes and cookies, and to enhance the flavor of desserts. To make an exquisite salad, pour a hazelnut-oil and lemon dressing over tender Boston head lettuce. The hazelnut oil makes this a crowning success.

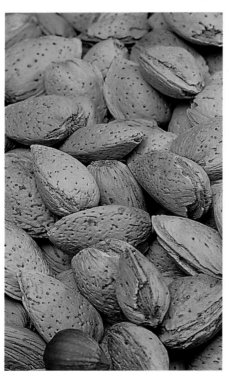

Almond Oil

Almond oil has been used for cosmetic purposes and as skin-friendly massage oil for many years, but it was only about twenty years ago that it was found to contain a good combination of fatty acids, which make it nutritionally valuable. There are sweet almonds and bitter almonds. Cold-pressed sweet almonds produce a pleasant-smelling and lightly flavored oil. Like olive oil, almond oil consists of mainly oleic acid (omega-9), which is a mono-unsaturated fatty acid and therefore fairly heat resistant. Almond oil is best used in baking pastries and cookies, but it also goes well with fish. Brush it on grilled plaice or trout towards the end of the cooking time or wrap it in foil and bake it in the oven.

Sesame Oil

Like most cooking oils on supermarket shelves, refined sesame oil is hexane extracted. There is also a roasted variety, which is dark brown in color with a strong smell and taste. These oils should be avoided as they are heavy in trans-fatty acids. However, some cold-pressed sesame oils have been introduced to the market recently. The oil is 46 percent mono-unsaturated (oleic) fatty acids, with 36 percent poly-unsaturated (linoleic) fatty acids. Cold-pressed sesame oil can be used in a variety of hot and cold dishes. It is especially useful in Asian recipes that call for sesame oil, and for sweet desserts. Sesame oil adds a distinct and pleasant flavor to hummus.

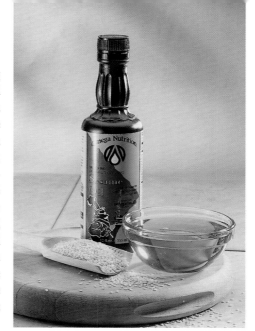

Pistachio Oil

This particularly fine culinary oil appeared on the culinary scene only in 1988 and therefore may be hard to find. Pistachio oil is dark green with a distinctive smell and taste. The nuts that are crushed for the oil come from Iran or Southern California. I rank pistachio oil as a highly nutritious and culinary oil, provided it is fresh and unrefined. Famous chefs have won medals and prizes preparing extraordinarily palatable dishes with pistachio oil. It goes well with pasta, and in dips and mayonnaise. When sauce and marinade recipes call for oil, try pistachio oil and be prepared for a surprise.

Pistachio oil has a pleasant, nutty aroma and a lingering, buttery-sweet taste. Its fatty acid profile shows 70 percent mono-unsaturated (oleic) fatty acids and 8 percent saturated (mainly palmitic) fatty acids. This means that pistachio oil can be heated to a medium heat of 160°C or 320°F.

Pistachio oil is usually sold in its natural, cold-processed, unrefined form and is available in most good health-food stores.

Avocado Oil

Avocados are often called "vegetarian butter." They are a highly nourishing food, which is rich in valuable fats. Interestingly, avocado oil is not cold pressed out of the fruit as the labels often

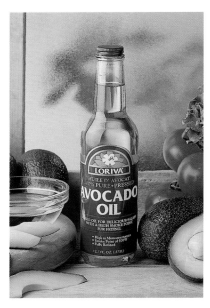

suggest, nor extracted with chemical solvents. Instead, mixing a paste of the ripe fruit with water and placing the mixture into a centrifuge produces a natural avocado oil. Avocado oil consists of 79 percent mono-unsaturated fatty acids, 16 percent saturated fatty acids and 5 percent poly-unsaturated fatty acids.

Kitchen tips for avocado oil

If you can find this wonderful oil, buy it. It has a discreet flavor that enhances the taste of both cold and hot dishes. Many fried foods, especially lean game meat, benefit from the flavor of this oil. Breakfast potatoes are a delicacy when fried in avocado oil. And once you have discovered the ease of making the best-tasting and healthiest mayonnaise from avocado oil, you will never go back to commercial brands.

Macadamia-Nut Oil

Macadamia nuts are native to Australia, where they are found in virtually every produce department. Rightfully called "the queen of nuts," macadamia nuts are 75 percent oil, which can be pressed into a true culinary oil.

Kitchen tips for macadamia-nut oil

Macadamia-nut oil is heat stable. Like avocado oil, it has a long shelf life because it consists of mostly mono-unsaturated and saturated fatty acids, which do not go rancid easily. The oil adds a fine, nutty flavor to many hot dishes, especially fish. Smoothies and desserts can be upgraded instantly with this oil.

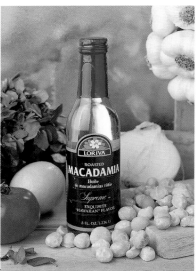

Coconut Oil or Coconut Butter

The coconut provides oil that is liquid in the countries where it is produced but solid in more temperate climates. From a chef who was born and raised in the tropics, but trained in exclusive hotels in Europe, I learned that coconut oil in its natural state is one of the best cooking oils. Coconuts and fish, as well as some other seafood, provide most of the nutritional fats consumed by people the world over. This chef made his own coconut cooking oil the same way indigenous peoples of tropical regions have done since time immemorial: by cracking open the hard shell of the coconut, scraping out the copra (as the nut flesh is called), and boiling it in water. The oil is then siphoned off as it floats to the top, and stored in bottles.

Coconut oil is widely and often exclusively used as a cooking oil by people in Madagascar, Indonesia, Malaysia, Vietnam, Sri Lanka and islanders in such places as Polynesia, the Philippines and the Caribbean. These people have exceedingly low rates of heart disease, no cholesterol problems and no clogged arteries. "These tropical oils have been consumed by many groups for thousands of years with absolutely no evidence of any harmful effects to the populations consuming them," says Dr. May Enig, PhD, the fats-and-oils expert who pulled the plug on margarine and other hydrogenated oils.

Coconut oil is 90 percent saturated fatty acids. However, these are lauric, myristic and palmitic fatty acids, which have low melting points. This is important because most of the satu-rates are in the form of medium chain triglycerides (MCTS),

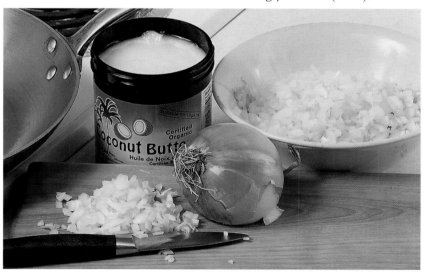

which are easily digested and not stored in the body as fat. In other words, you will not gain weight by eating coconut oil. Other good fatty acids in coconut oil are 7.5 percent mono-unsaturated oleic fatty acids and 2.5% poly-unsaturated linoleic fatty acids.

What Natural, Unrefined Coconut Oil Does *Not* Do

Natural, unrefined coconut oil should be recognized mainly for what it doesn't do.
- it does *not* raise cholesterol
- it does *not* clog arteries
- it does *not* cause coronary heart disease
- it does *not* cause obesity by depositing calories as body fat

Unprocessed Coconut Oil Has Many Health Benefits

- it contains a component that is anti-microbial and anti-viral and thus it kills germs
- it protects users from tropical parasites and infections
- it contains easily digested MTFS, which help people who have problems absorbing conventional fats
- as one of a very few plants containing lauric acid (MCT), also found in human breast milk, it can be a lifesaver for premature babies

Kitchen tips for coconut oil

Coconut oil is one of the best oils for cooking, baking and frying, but be sure you are using it in its natural, unhydrogenated form. This is sold in health-food stores and can be recognized by its off-white to grayish-yellow color. The label should say "unrefined." It is a stable oil with a long shelf life and very useful in a whole-foods kitchen. Its melting point is 23-26°C, depending on its country of origin. Therefore it can be whipped up for use in pie crusts, cookies, muffins, breads or cakes. Use it in any recipe or for anything that calls for lard or vegetable shortening. Coconut butter adds a nice flavor to stir fries and sautéed vegetables. Dr. Budwig has shared with us her recipe for butter blended with coconut butter as a healthy substitute for margarine (see page 46).

Other Oils

A number of other vegetable oils are popular in the market place and sold in huge quantities in supermarkets and groceries. These commercial oils include sunflower, safflower, peanut, corn, soya and canola oils, all of which are made from the seeds of genetically engineered plants. Most are hexane-extracted or, if expeller-pressed, are refined at high heats and treated with chemicals. In addition, they are packaged in white plastics bottles, not protected from light and often contain significant amounts of trans-fatty acids. The manufacturers do not reveal their fatty-acid profiles, but a test sponsored by *alive* magazine showed that one brand of canola oil contained 3.5 percent trans-fatty acids.

Canola Oil is a fairly recent newcomer on the market. It has gained popularity for two reasons: First because of a well funded advertising campaign tauting it as a "heart healthy" oil, and second because of its low price, by which it has gained a huge market share at the cost of safflower, corn and sunflower oils.

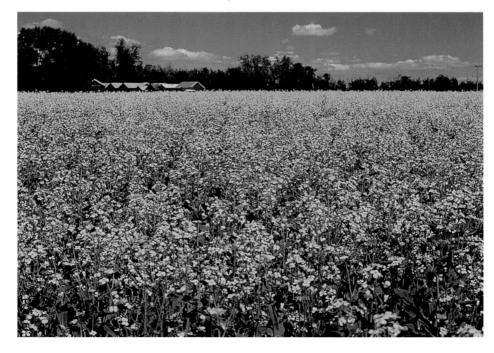

Canola oil is the product of genetically engineered rape seeds. Rape seed oil is unsuited for human consumption because it contains erucic acid, a very long chain fatty acid which can cause fibrotic heart lesions. By modifying the rape seeds it was hoped to create an oil rich in healthy fatty acids. However, in the refining and deodorizing process, which is done with high heat (450° to 500° F), some of the good fats are turned into trans-fatty acids (bad fats). Recent studies also show that refined canola oil actually causes a deficiency in vitamin E, a vitamin required for a healthy heart, and traces of the erucic acid that causes heart lesions, especially when the diet is low in saturated fats. Canola oil and other refined oils have no place in a whole-foods kitchen, as they have been stripped of all valuable life elements and contain dangerous fats as a result of processing.

Head to your local health food store to purchase healthy alternatives to supermarket oils. They are good, healthy oils with rich color and strong taste. The higher price is well worth the price of your health. Cutting out processed fats and oils and replacing them with unrefined oils will bring you better health.

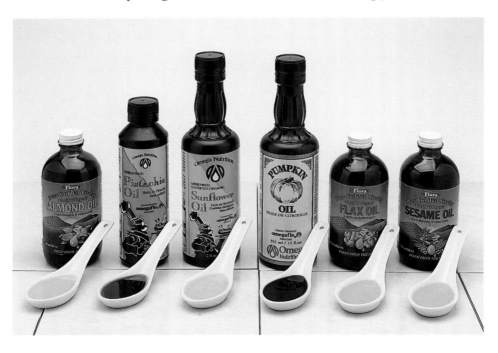

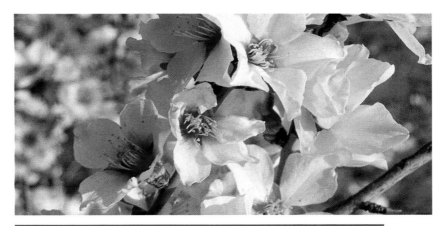

Unrefined Oils Listed by Heat Tolerance

Below is a list of the unrefined oils described in this volume, which you can use for cooking, baking and stir frying. They are listed in descending order from the most heat tolerant to the least.

Natural Oil	Smoke Point
Coconut Oil	230°C
Almond Oil	220°C
Avocado Oil	220°C
Macadamia-nut Oil	200°C
Olive Oil	190°C
Sunflower Oil	170°C
Safflower Oil	160°C
Hazelnut Oil	150°C
Sesame Oil	150°C
DO NOT heat the following oils at all:	
Pumpkinseed Oil	112°C
Walnut Oil	112°C
Flax Oil	112°C

The lower the smoke point, the easier it is to damage fatty acids. To avoid overheating, perform the following test:

Heat the oil. Then take a slice of onion and dip it in the hot oil. When the oil sizzles, it is hot enough for frying. Do not raise the oil temperature higher as you might reach the smoke point, which is when the oil becomes toxic trans-fatty acids are formed. If the oil does reach the smoking point by accident, throw it out, wash your pan and start over again.

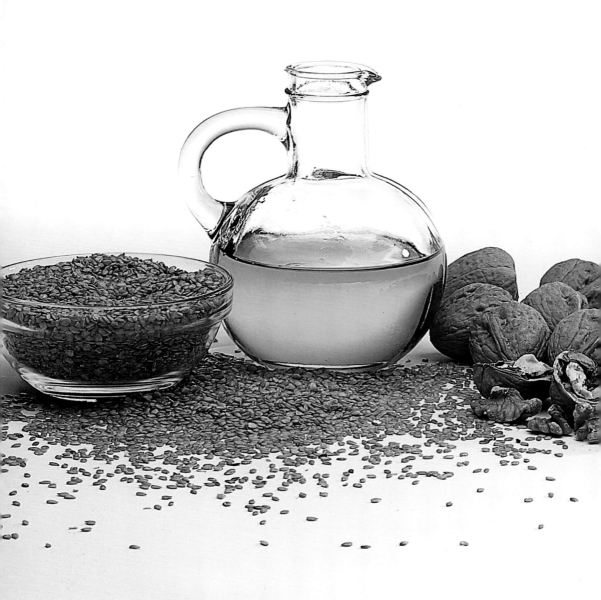

Healthy Recipes Using Good Fats and Oils

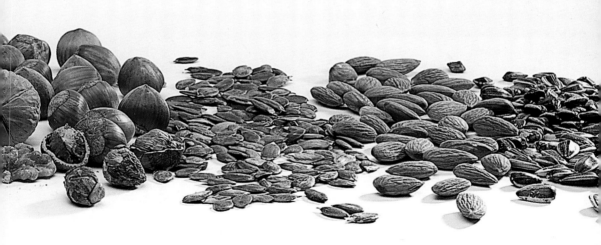

Researchers are only beginning to discover the many good elements that fats contribute to health. Take advantage of these elements by preparing healthful meals with good fats and oils.

Quark with Flax Oil

This traditional East German specialty is a tastier and healthier version of sour cream. It is delicious when served with baked potatoes, steamed carrots or corn. You can even carry it to work in a container and spread it on fresh rye bread, Swedish crisp bread or a cold baked potato.

I cup quark

4 tbsp flax oil

Herb seasoning salt to taste

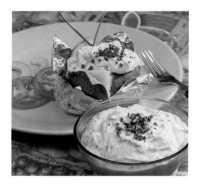

Variation 1: Season the quark with fresh, finely chopped dill—the more dill, the better the flavor—or add a generous amount of finely chopped chives to the quark for a surprisingly gratifying meal!

Variation 2: Grate fresh horseradish and mix it into the quark. The taste will be a surprise for your palate and the horseradish will act as an antibiotic for the urinary tract and kidney, and will even ease bladder discomfort.

Kefir Quark with Flax Oil Dip

For a party lunch you may want to surprise your guests with this delicious new dip.

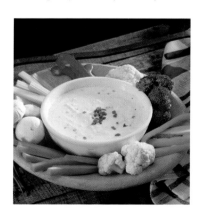

To make kefir quark simply pour kefir into a jar and place the jar in a pot of boiling water until the milk solids separate from the whey. Pour through a fine mesh strainer or cheesecloth and let stand overnight. The next morning you will have fresh tasting creamy cheese known as quark.

Then, add a few tablespoons of kefir to the recipe above. Add crushed garlic to taste. Serve with tomatoes, radishes, celery, carrots, broccoli or any other vegetables.

Variation: If you don't want to make kefir, use natural plain yogurt or buttermilk instead.

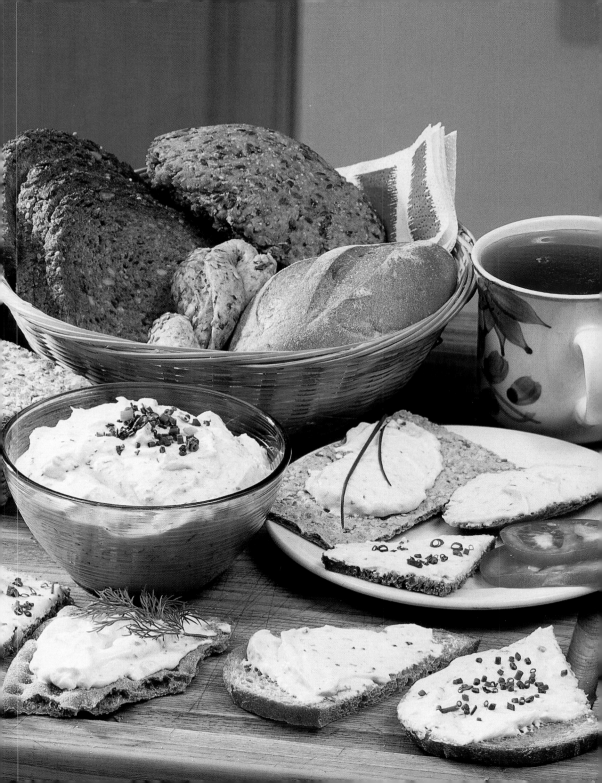

Coconut Butter Bread Spread

Many people want a tasty alternative to butter. I have experimented with a blend of coconut butter and flax oil and found it makes an extraordinary sandwich spread—especially with the addition of sautéed onions. The spread, if kept refrigerated, will stay fresh for several months.

1¼ cups coconut butter

2 large onions, finely chopped

1 tsp sea salt

1 cup (250 ml) **flax oil**

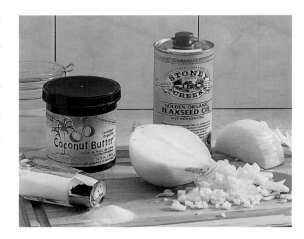

Try this spread on fresh rye bread with herbal salt. You'll love it.

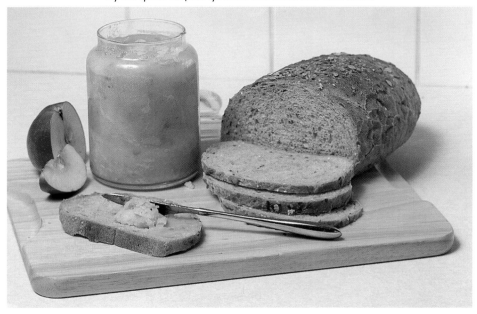

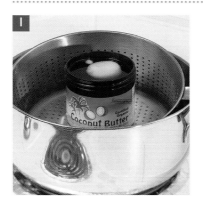

1 Place the coconut butter in a small container then set the container in a large bowl of warm water. This will soften the coconut butter and make it easier to work with. Be careful not to let the water run over the sides of the container.

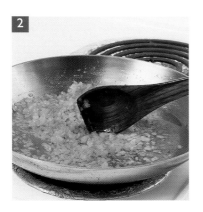

2 Pour ⅓ of the melted coconut butter into a saucepan over medium heat. Add chopped onion and salt and sauté, stirring constantly with a wooden spatula until the onions start to brown. Turn the heat down to low and carefully sauté the onions for a few more seconds without burning them.

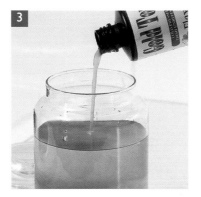

3 Remove from the heat, let cool to room temperature and then mix with the remaining coconut butter and the cold refrigerated flax oil. Pour into a container, seal tightly and place in the refrigerator. Turn the container upside down every ten minutes or stir the spread to prevent the onions from sinking to the bottom.

Classic Flax Oil Dressing

The most important ingredient in a salad dressing is the natural, unrefined fresh oil, such as flax, walnut, hazelnut or pumpkin seed oil. This classic recipe is wonderful on top of tender leaf lettuce or finely grated carrots.

4 tbsp flax seed oil

Juice of I lemon

I tsp Maggi, soy sauce or Bragg's aminos

2 tbsp onion, minced

Green onions, chopped (optional)

½ tsp mixed dry salad herbs

In a bowl, beat lemon juice and flax seed oil until creamy. Stir in the Maggi and onions and add the herbs.

Serves 4

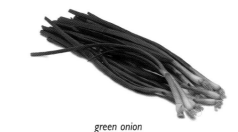

green onion

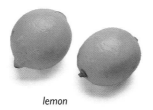

lemon

Good fats make meals tasty and more importantly prevent overeating as they give you a sense of satisfaction. Fat-free diets don't satisfy hunger and lead to snacking, which results in obesity.

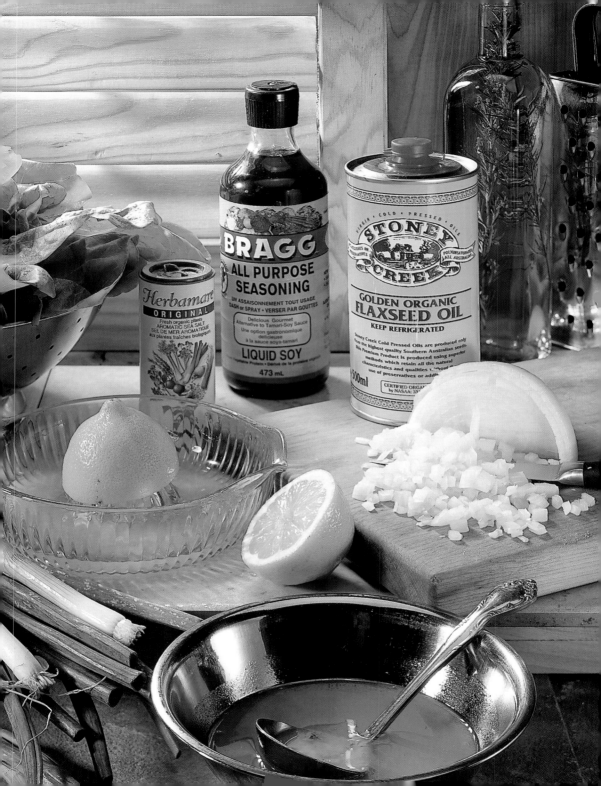

Walnut or Hazelnut Oil Dressing

Create an amazingly delicious and simple salad dressing in a jiffy with just these few ingredients.

3 tbsp walnut or hazelnut oil

Juice of 1 lemon

Spritzer Maggi or Bragg's aminos

Pinch celery salt or herbal salt (such as Herbamare), **to taste**

In a bowl, whisk together all the ingredients.

Serves 2

Variations:

Add one or all of these ingredients:

1 clove garlic

⅛ tsp Dijon mustard

1 small onion, finely chopped

1 tsp organic maple syrup

Freshly ground pepper, to taste

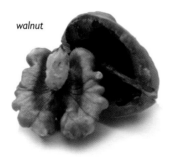

walnut

This dressing is especially suited for the tender salad leaves of Boston head lettuce or lime stone lettuce. And if you ever find corn salad, also called lamb's quarters, rapunzel, field lettuce or mâché, use hazelnut oil exclusively.

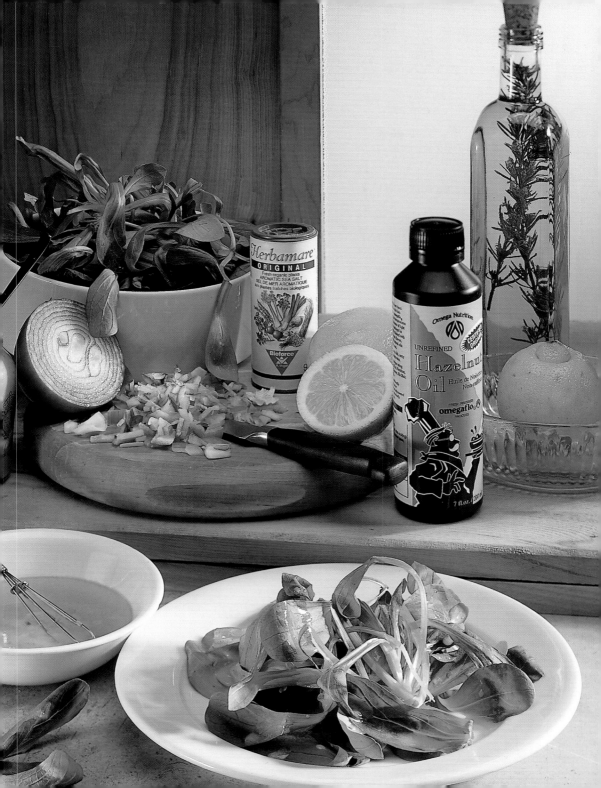

Roquefort Cheese Dressing with Pumpkin Seed Oil

A cheese dressing requires a more robust leafy lettuce, such as romaine, endive or French crisp batavia lettuce.

4 tbsp genuine Roquefort cheese

4 tbsp pumpkin seed oil

½ cup (125 ml) kefir or sour cream

Juice of 1 lemon

1 tsp Maggi or Bragg's aminos

1 tbsp red or white wine vinegar or Molkosan

½ tsp dried Italian herbs

1 clove garlic, minced

Place all ingredients in a bowl and blend with a hand mixer.

This will make a very smooth and delicious cheese dressing. If you prefer chunks of cheese in the dressing, reserve half the cheese and crumble it in before serving.

Serves 4

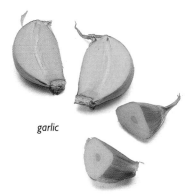

garlic

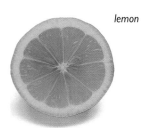

lemon

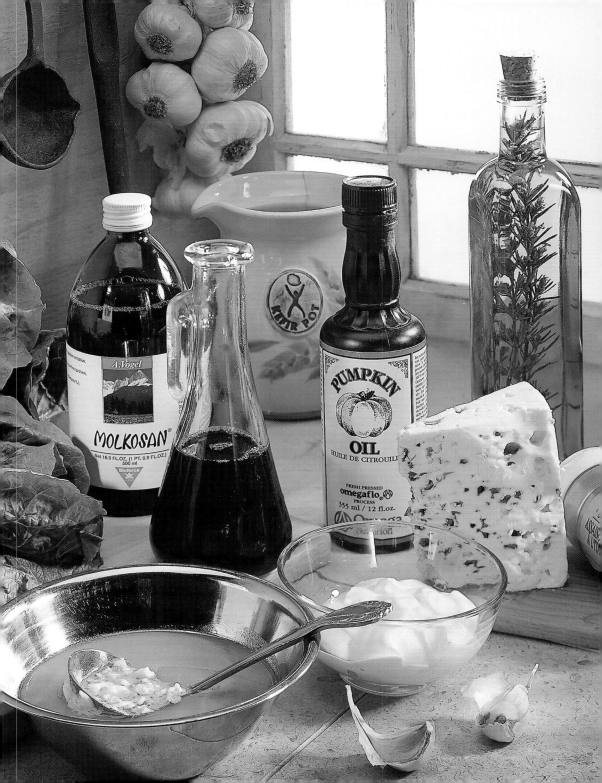

Potato Salad with Pumpkin Seed Oil

This potato salad is always a big hit at *alive* company functions.

1½ lbs (750 g) yellow salad potatoes

1 vegetable bouillon cube

4 tbsp hot water

4 tbsp pumpkin seed oil

Juice of 1 lemon

1 medium onion, finely chopped

1 dill pickle, finely chopped

Pinch Herbamare seasoning, to taste (or chives, parsley or fresh dill, finely cut)

2 large free-range eggs, soft-boiled and sliced

Boil the potatoes until tender then drain and let cool. Slice the potatoes ¼" (5 mm) thick.

In a large bowl, dissolve the vegetable bouillon in hot water. Add oil, lemon juice, onion, pickle and seasoning; mix thoroughly. Gently mix in potatoes and eggs and serve.

Serves 4

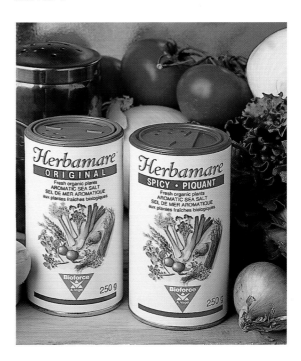

To soft boil the eggs, bring a small pot of water to a boil and add the eggs slowly with a large spoon. Cook for exactly 7 minutes then remove from heat, drain the water and rinse eggs under cold water. Crack the top of the eggs immediately to prevent them from cooking any longer. The yolks should be slightly runny.

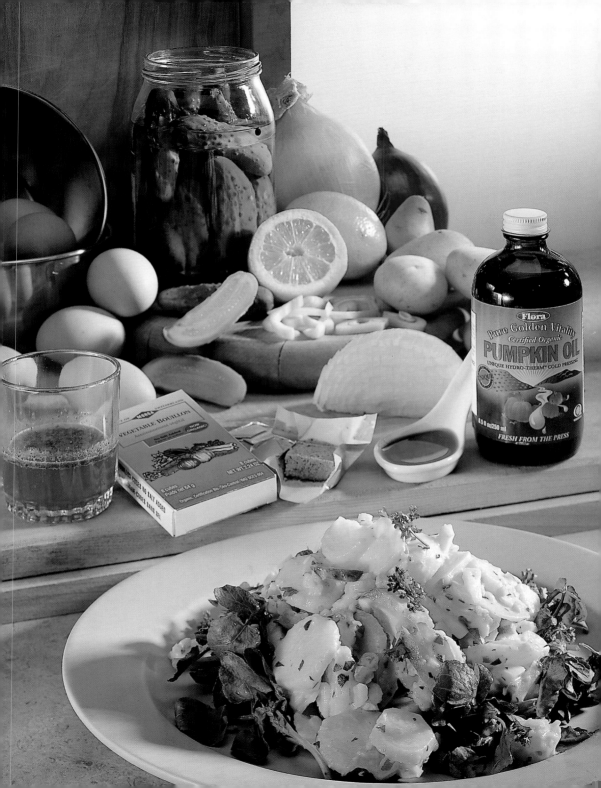

Green Mayonnaise

The key to this recipe is to add the kefir last as the crowning touch. This light mayonnaise is easily digested and leaves a good feeling in your stomach.

½ **cup** (125 ml) **pumpkin seed oil**

1 **egg yolk**

1 **tsp Dijon mustard**

1 **clove garlic, minced**

Sea salt and freshly ground pepper, to taste

½ **cup** (125 ml) **kefir** (or natural yogurt or sour cream)

In a bowl, blend all ingredients with a hand mixer, adding kefir last, until mixture is creamy. Use in any recipe calling for mayonnaise–with eggs, vegetables, as dip or salad dressing.

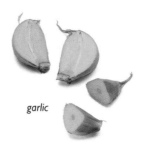

garlic

Pumpkin Seed Oil Dressing

This dressing is a simple delicacy suitable for most green salads, Boston head or loose-leaf lettuce, endive, romaine, radicchio, arugula or even wild greens.

3 **tbsp pumpkin seed oil**

Juice of 1 lemon

Dash fine balsamic vinegar

Dash Maggi, soya sauce or Bragg's aminos

⅛ **tsp Herbamare seasoning** (about 4 shakes)

In a bowl, whisk together all ingredients until creamy. Pour over greens and serve immediately.

Makes 4-6 servings

> What about a colorful green potato salad? It may look different–but wait 'til you taste it.

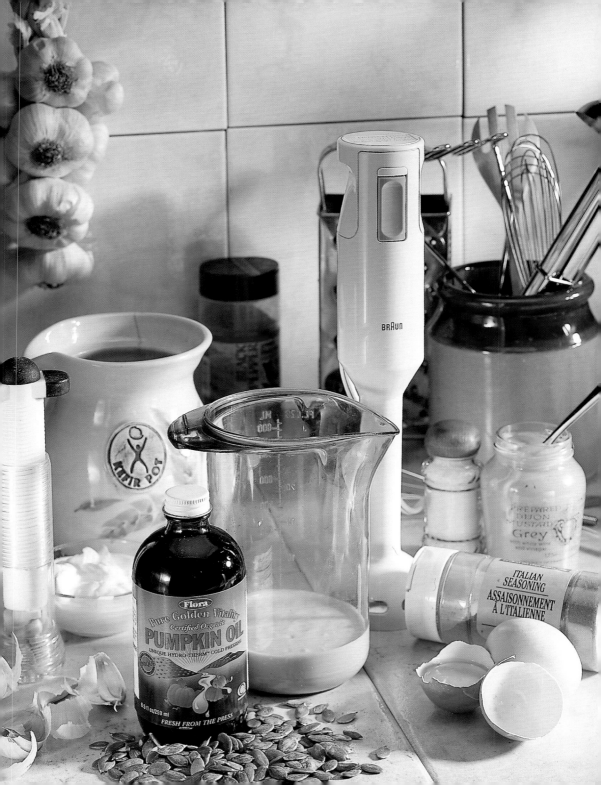

Chèvre à l'Huile (Goat Cheese in Olive Oil)

When you want to impress unexpected guests, serve this quick and easy dish and you'll have them dropping by more often! It surprises the palate and tastes excellent with a crisp salad or on toasted rye bread.

1 lb (500 g) **young goat cheese or Feta cheese, cut in 1"** (2.5 cm) **slices**

5 sprigs fresh herbs, use 1 each or a mix of thyme, basil, tarragon or oregano

2 bay leaves

1 dozen black peppercorns

1 large clove garlic, quartered

2 cups (500 ml) **extra-virgin olive oil**

In a 1-quart (1-liter) airtight screw top glass container, layer the cheese alternatively with the herbs, peppercorns and garlic. Fill the container with oil and close tightly.

Store the container in a cool place, for 1 to 2 weeks to mature, then store in the refrigerator. Use a clean fork each time you take out some cheese to prevent bacteria from entering the container. Keep lid tightly closed. The cheese will keep for up to 10 weeks, but I bet you it won't last that long; it tastes too good.

The best goat's cheese comes in a roll.

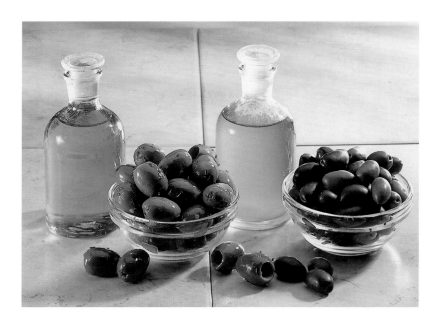

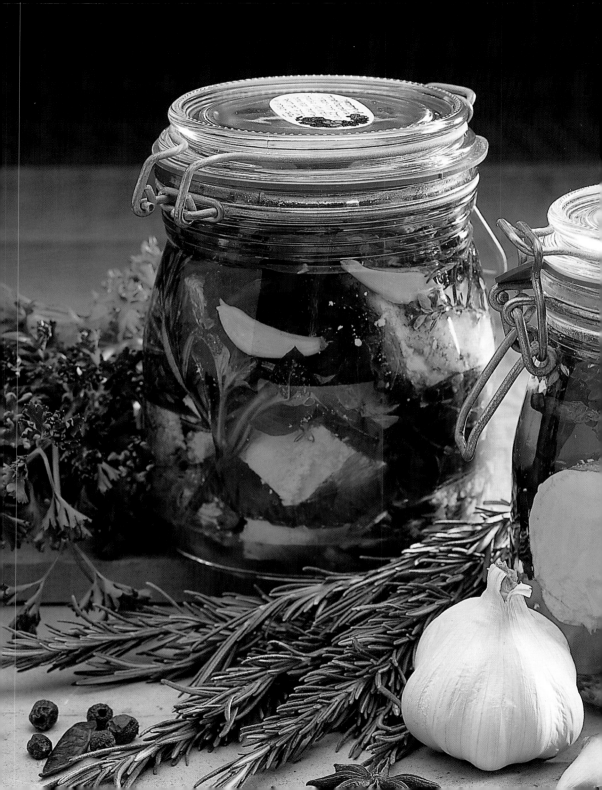

Potato Pancakes with Coconut Oil

Serve this quick and easy dish with a leafy green salad for a satisfying meal.

4 large potatoes, peeled and finely grated

1 medium-size onion, diced

1 free-range egg

½ tsp sea salt

1 tsp Maggi or Bragg's aminos

2 tbsp coconut butter

In a bowl, combine all ingredients, except the coconut butter. In a large frying pan, heat 1 tablespoon of coconut butter over medium heat. When the coconut butter is melted and hot, place 4 heaping tablespoons of pancake mixture in the pan and flatten them with a spatula. Fry until both sides are golden brown. Repeat until all batter is gone, making sure that the next tablespoon of coconut butter heats up before adding the pancake batter.

Serves 4

Greek Salad with Olive Oil

You'll find this traditional salad on the menu of all Greek restaurants. It's easy to prepare and a refreshing whole foods addition to any meal.

3 ripe tomatoes, diced

½ English cucumber, diced

1 cup (250 ml) **Feta cheese, crumbled**

20 Kalamata olives

A few capers

1 tbsp fresh oregano, finely cut

1 tsp balsamic vinegar

5 tbsp extra-virgin olive oil

1 tbsp red onions, cut in half rings or diced

Sea salt and freshly ground pepper, to taste

In a large bowl, thoroughly combine all ingredients.

Serves 4

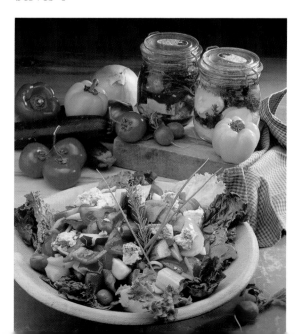

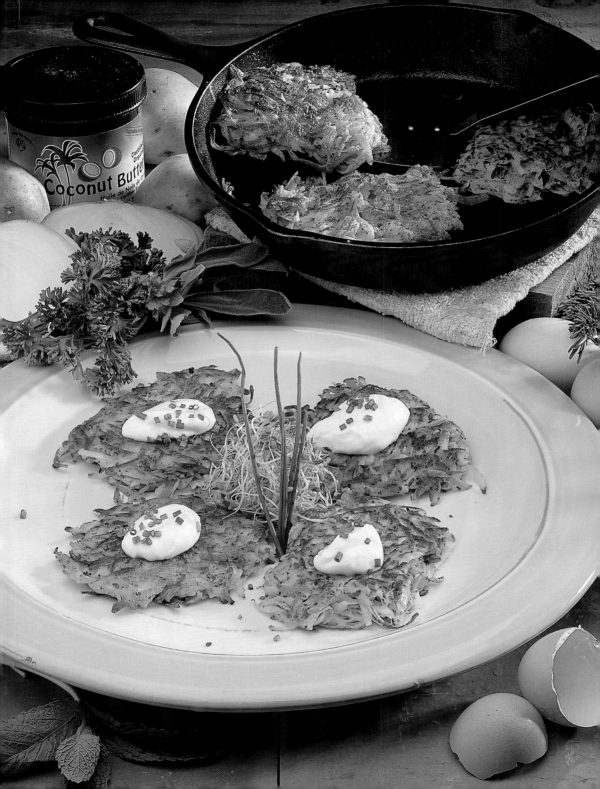

Marinade for Fish

Use any of these oils for the marinade: avocado, macadamia nut, almond, coconut or olive oil. When cooked on low heat, these oils magically create a crispy outside, without burning the fat or the protein, and enhance flavor immensely.

3 tbsp avocado oil (or macadamia, almond, coconut or olive oil)

2 tbsp Dijon mustard

1 tbsp freshly ground pepper

2 cloves garlic, minced

In a bowl, combine oil and mustard then stir in pepper and garlic. Brush the marinade on the fish of your choice and panfry on low heat.

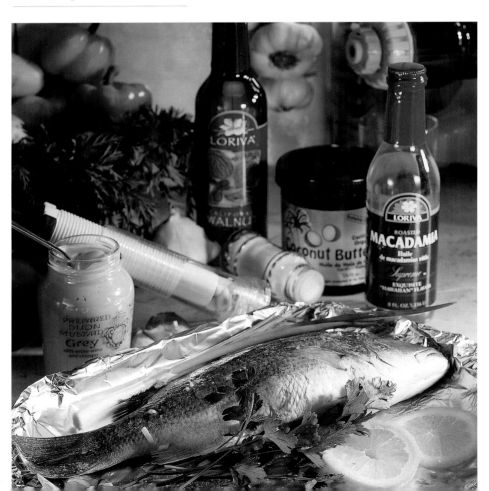

Baked Biscuits with Almond Oil

This light sweet-tooth delicacy goes well with an afternoon coffee, or served with vanilla ice cream and fresh strawberries.

3 free-range eggs

4 tbsp Sucanat or Rapadura (dried cane juice sugar)

4 tsp almond oil (or extra-virgin olive oil or coconut butter)

4 tbsp sweet white wine

I cup (200 g) **whole wheat flour**

I tsp baking powder

Pinch sea salt

I tbsp butter or coconut butter, to grease pan

Nutmeg, freshly grated, for garnish (optional)

Preheat oven to 400°F (200°C).

For biscotti: In a large bowl, beat eggs and sugar using a hand mixer. Stir in oil and wine, then sift in the flour, baking powder and salt. Mix until the dough is smooth. Pour the dough into a butter-greased springform pan and bake for 35 to 40 minutes. Cool for 5 minutes then slice.

For a real treat, sprinkle lightly with freshly grated nutmeg and serve warm.

For cookies: Follow above directions and spoon cookie balls from dough. Bake for 35 to 40 minutes.

Baking with natural unrefined oils, such as almond and hazelnut, adds both taste and nutrition to baked treats.

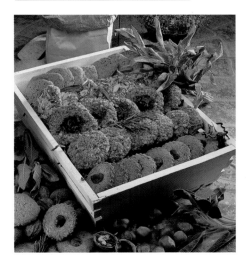

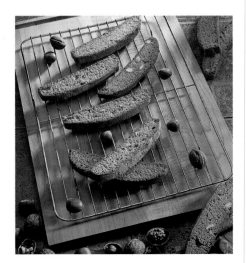

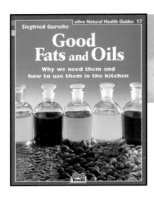

alive Natural Health Guides 17
Siegfried Gursche

Good Fats and Oils

Why we need them and
how to use them in the kitchen

books

Natural
Your best source of

We hope you enjoyed **Good Fats and Oils**.
There are 31 other titles to choose from in *alive*'s library
of Natural Health Guides, and more coming soon. The first
series of its kind in North America - now sold on 5 continents!

Self-Help Information

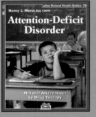
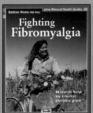
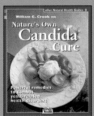
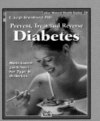
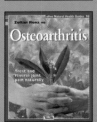
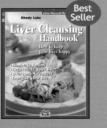
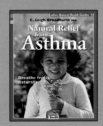
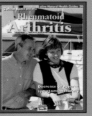

Healing Foods & Herbs

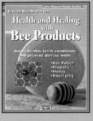
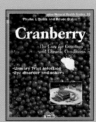
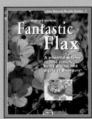
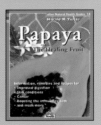
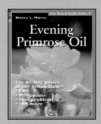
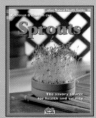
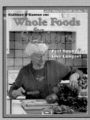
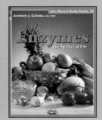

expert authors   easy-to-read information   tasty recipes